Trim and Thrive

A Blueprint for Sustainable Weight Loss

Rossana Lewis

Email: rossanalewis01@gmail.com

TABLE OF CONTENT

Chapter 1: Understanding Weight Loss Essentials

1.1 Demystifying Weight Loss Strategies

Weight loss is a complex physiological process that involves a delicate balance between calorie intake and energy expenditure. In a world where fad diets and quick fixes abound, it's essential to understand the science behind weight loss to make informed decisions about our health. This article aims to demystify the mechanics of weight loss, exploring the fundamental principles that drive this transformative journey.

The Caloric Equation

At the core of weight loss lies the concept of the energy balance equation. This equation compares the calories consumed through food and beverages to the calories expended through basal metabolic rate (BMR)—the energy required for basic bodily functions and physical activity. When you consume more calories than you expend, the surplus is stored as fat, leading to weight gain. Conversely, a calorie deficit, where expenditure exceeds intake, prompts the body to use stored fat for energy, resulting in weight loss.

Metabolism's Role

Metabolism, the intricate process by which the body converts food into energy, plays a pivotal role in weight loss. A higher metabolic rate burns more calories even at rest, aiding in weight loss efforts. Factors influencing metabolism include genetics, muscle mass, age, and hormonal fluctuations. Muscle tissue consumes more energy than fat, so incorporating strength training into your routine can boost metabolism and aid in sustainable weight loss.

Nutrition's Impact

Diet plays a crucial role in weight loss success. Consuming nutrient-dense, whole foods like fruits, vegetables, lean proteins, and whole grains helps control calorie intake while providing essential nutrients for optimal bodily function. Avoiding overly restrictive diets is important, as they may lead to nutrient deficiencies and metabolic slowdown. Portion control, mindful eating, and reducing the consumption of processed and sugary foods contribute to healthier weight loss.

Exercise and Activity

Regular physical activity not only burns calories but also enhances weight loss by preserving muscle mass and improving metabolic efficiency. Cardiovascular exercises like running, swimming, and cycling burn calories directly, while strength training builds muscle, increasing overall calorie expenditure. A combination of both types of exercise is ideal for balanced and effective weight loss.

The Role of Hormones

Hormones play a significant role in regulating appetite, metabolism, and fat storage. Hormonal imbalances, often associated with conditions like hypothyroidism or polycystic ovary syndrome (PCOS), can hinder weight loss efforts. Consulting a healthcare professional to address hormonal concerns is crucial for those facing such challenges.

The journey to weight loss should prioritize sustainability and health over rapid results. Crash diets and extreme restrictions can lead to muscle loss, nutrient deficiencies, and a rebound in weight. Slow and steady weight loss, aiming for 1–2 pounds per week, is more likely to yield lasting results.

1.2 Embracing Sustainable Approaches

So, you've decided to take charge of your weight and become a fitter version of yourself. That's commendable! But let's keep it real – the road to weight loss can be a bit rocky. It requires dedication, persistence, and a basic understanding of nutrition.

Initially, you might be a bit overwhelmed since the weight loss space is a bit different from what you're used to, but if you're on a sustainable diet, you'll get used to it with time and start to enjoy it.

Let's take a quick look at things you need to do to lose weight sustainably:

Set Realistic Goals: You may be tempted to achieve your dream body in a flash, but you must slow down if you'll lose weight in a sustainable way. Findings from research show that losing 1-2 pounds per week is a healthy and attainable target. Anything beyond this may disrupt your body's metabolic processes. You have to apply the same SMART rule that you use to achieve other goals to your body goals. By setting specific, measurable, achievable, realistic, and time-bound body goals, you can avoid feelings of frustration and disappointment accompanying unrealistic goals. Quickly grab a pen and write out your SMART body goals!

- Specific: Instead of saying, 'I want to shed some weight,' switch to 'I want to lose 10 kilograms (22 pounds) of my body weight'. That is specific; you can write that down and put it anywhere where it's easy to see. Aim for a gradual and steady weight loss of 0.5 to 1 kg (1 to 2 pounds) per week, which is generally considered sustainable and healthier.

- Measurable: How will you track your progress? Will you weigh yourself weekly? Keep a food diary? Stick to small portion sizes of foods? Avoid processed foods. Avoid alcohol or reduce it to 1 glass per week. Write down the changes you want to measure to ensure success.

- Achievable: It's crucial to set goals and strategies that will challenge you slightly but within reach. For instance, Based on a safe and sustainable rate of weight loss, I will lose 5 to 1 kilogram per week, which is achievable. Also, check your strategies. Can you exercise 1 hour daily to achieve weight loss, or 45mins is more possible? Find a realistic balance that will challenge you but also be achievable.

- Relevant: Are your weight loss goals relevant to your health or just the dress size? While dress size is valid, it could put you under unnecessary pressure, especially if the dress you're trying to fit into is way small. But when you set body weight goals relevant to your health, it takes the pressure off you. For example, 'I want to lose weight to increase my energy level, be more flexible, and reduce my risk of chronic conditions.

- Time-bound: It's essential to set a timeframe for your goals. Break down your main goal of losing 10 kg into smaller milestones with specific completion dates. For example, You already set 0.5-1kg per week. How long will it take to lose 10kg? That's like 10 weeks if you stick to your measurable strategies.

Let's put it all together: "I will lose 10 kilograms (22 pounds) of body weight within 10 weeks by reducing my portion of meals, avoiding sodas, and engaging in regular physical activity. I will track my progress by weighing myself weekly, keeping a food diary, and adjusting my approach as needed."

Navigate Emotional Eating: Emotional eating is that sneaky villain that tries to hijack your progress. We've all been there; Stress, boredom, or sadness can make you crave food like never before. Research suggests that emotional eating is associated with greater body mass index (BMI) and poorer weight loss outcomes. It's like a lightbulb moment when people realize,' I eat even when I am not really hungry!'
How do you intend to overcome the emotional triggers that cause you to overeat? You can take a walk, remove junk from your refrigerator and stick with fruits and veggies, jot down your

thoughts, or chat with a friend. Once you release the emotions tied to overeating, you'll experience the freedom to make healthier food choices.

Build a Healthy Plate: Now, let's talk about constructing a plate that screams balance. Imagine your plate as a canvas, and you're the artist. You can control calorie intake by prioritizing nutrient-dense foods while ensuring optimal nutrition. Fill half of your plate with non-starchy vegetables like ugwu, kale, broccoli, spinach, or peppers, as they are low in calories and high in fiber, aiding in satiety. Let a quarter of your plate be for lean protein sources, such as chicken, fish, or tofu, which can help preserve muscle mass during weight loss. The remaining quarter should be for whole grains like quinoa or brown rice, providing sustained energy and essential nutrients.

Mindful Eating: Practicing mindful eating can transform your relationship with food and support weight loss efforts. Research indicates that mindfulness-based interventions can reduce emotional eating. How do you practice mindful eating? Chew slowly and savor each bite, paying attention to flavors and textures. Tune in to your body's hunger and fullness cues. Eat when you're truly hungry, and stop eating when you feel comfortably satisfied. Avoid distractions like television or smartphones during meals, which can lead to mindless overeating. By being present and aware, you'll be more in tune with your body's signals of fullness and satisfaction.

Stay Active: Regular physical activity is essential for weight loss and overall well-being. Engaging in both cardiovascular (aerobic) exercises and strength training can help you burn calories, build lean muscle mass, and increase metabolism. Aim for at least 150 minutes of moderate-intensity exercise per week. Find activities you enjoy, such as walking, cycling, dancing, or swimming, and incorporate strength training exercises to further enhance your weight loss efforts.

Chapter 2: Building Your Nutrition Foundation

2.1 Essential Nutrients for Weight Loss

What actually contributes to your weight loss are some of the nutrients that are found in food. Following a diet based on your own food preferences and adopting a nutrient guideline is what is necessary to achieve your weight loss goal. Recommendations for carbohydrates, protein and fat depend on your total calorie intake during the weight loss process. Many adults don't get enough of nutrients that are necessary to attain a healthy weight loss goal. Losing weight isn't just about cutting calories, as a low-calorie diet can do more harm than good if you aren't getting the right amount of nutrients.

Below are some of the nutrients to lose weight:
Arginine: Research has found that administering arginine to obese women over 12 weeks resulted in a 3-inch average reduction in waist size and a 6.5-pound average weight loss.

Magnesium: This mineral helps in burning of the fat. Higher magnesium intake was associated with lower levels of fasting glucose and insulin, as noted by a popular study.

Potassium: Potassium helps in flattening your belly and also aids with muscle recovery after a workout. It also helps reduce bloat by flushing out the excess sodium from the body.

Choline: This is a fat-blasting B vitamin that turns off the genes that cause your body to store fat around your liver. Make sure to include this nutrient on a daily basis.

Resistant Starch: Also known as slow carbs, resistant starch passes through the small intestine without being digested. It feeds on the healthy gut bacteria that helps you keep yourself fuller for longer and burns fat.

Omega-3 Fatty Acids: Omega-3 FAs help reduce the stomach fat storage by dealing with inflammation. Further, it was also found that people with highest levels of omega-3s lived two years longer than those who didn't. This is one of the best nutrients to lose weight.

Leucine: This amino acid increases the body's ability to synthesize protein. It helps in reducing body fat and also in maintaining a lean body mass.

Vitamin D: This vitamin helps in regulating the appetite. This vitamin has to be a part of your weight loss diet and it particularly helps in reducing the fat from your belly area.

Monounsaturated Fats: These healthy fats prevent the storage of belly flubber. It was found that those who ate half a fresh avocado, which is rich in oleic acid, reported a 40% decrease in the desire to eat for hours afterwards.

Calcium: Calcium helps your body burn more fat. It also maintains your energy levels of the body and you wouldn't get the desire to rush to a bag of chips due to hunger later on. This is one of the best nutrients to lose weight.

Vitamin C: Stress is caused by high levels of cortisol that causes belly fat storage. Vitamin C is an antioxidant that has been proven to help people cope with stress and hence prevent weight gain.

Selenium: Those people with a sluggish thyroid gland exhibit deficiencies in selenium along with slowed metabolism and weight gain. A supplementation of 80 micrograms of selenium per day will help reduce anti-thyroid antibodies.

B Vitamins: Vitamin B12 helps to metabolize two main energy sources, which are fats and carbohydrates. This is one of the best nutrients that is required to lose weight.

Tryptophan: Getting good sleep helps us lose weight. It helps our body recover and also builds muscle mass. If you're not getting good sleep, then you must go for food sources of amino acid - tryptophan, which is a precursor to serotonin. This gets converted to melatonin to encourage sleep. This is one of the best nutrients to lose weight.

2.2 Crafting Your Personalized Meal Plan

In the quest for weight loss, one-size-fits-all approaches often fall short of expectations. The key to achieving sustainable and effective weight loss lies in a personalized meal plan. Let's explore the significance of a personalized meal plan for weight loss and guide you on how to create one that suits your unique needs.

Assessing Your Current Lifestyle and Goals: To craft a personalized meal plan, begin by assessing your current lifestyle and setting clear weight loss goals. Are you looking to shed pounds rapidly or adopt a more gradual, sustainable approach? Understanding your goals and your daily routine will help determine the right caloric intake and macronutrient distribution.

Identifying Your Nutritional Needs: Once you've defined your goals, it's essential to identify your nutritional needs. Are you dealing with any specific dietary restrictions, allergies, or intolerances? Consider any medical conditions that might impact your food choices. This information will help you create a meal plan that not only supports weight loss but also caters to your overall well-being.

Balancing Macronutrients: Effective weight loss meal plans should strike a balance between macronutrients: carbohydrates, proteins, and fats. The distribution of these nutrients in your diet is crucial for managing hunger, stabilizing blood sugar levels, and promoting fat loss. Depending on your goals, you can tailor your macronutrient ratios accordingly.

Portion Control and Caloric Intake: Portion control plays a vital role in weight loss. By controlling the number of calories you consume, you can create a calorie deficit necessary for losing weight. Ensure that your meal plan includes appropriate serving sizes to meet your caloric goals.

Meal Frequency and Timing: The timing of your meals can affect your metabolism and energy levels. Some individuals benefit from frequent, smaller meals, while others prefer intermittent fasting. A personalized meal plan should align with your preferences and daily schedule.

Choosing Nutrient-Dense Foods: A well-balanced meal plan should include nutrient-dense foods that provide essential vitamins, minerals, and antioxidants. Focus on incorporating whole grains, lean proteins, healthy fats, and a variety of fruits and vegetables into your diet.

Staying Hydrated: Proper hydration is often overlooked but is a crucial aspect of a personalized meal plan for weight loss. Water supports metabolism, aids in digestion, and can help control appetite. Ensure that you're drinking enough water throughout the day.

Monitoring Progress and Adjusting Your Plan: Creating a personalized meal plan for weight loss is not a one-time task. Regularly monitor your progress and be prepared to adjust your plan as needed. Your body's response to dietary changes may require modifications to your meal plan, ensuring that it remains effective over time.

Chapter 3: Meal Prep and Recipes

3.1 Meal Preparation Techniques

Have a Plan: The first rule of meal prepping is to plan ahead. It doesn't help to meal prep if you don't know what exactly you're preparing and why. So think about the types of meals that you want to cook and the types of recipes you're good at preparing, and make sure to come up with a versatile meal plan that you can use as your go-to for a number of months.

Another helpful element of meal prepping is to plan your meal times in advance. Instead of eating haphazardly or when you feel the urge, designate specific meal times and stick to them. Not only will this prevent unwanted and unplanned indulgence in unhealthy snacks, but it'll also reduce those midsection inches and keep you healthier.

Create a Grocery Shopping List: Once you've figured out what you'll be eating and when now it's time to go shopping. The trick to sticking to your planned meals is to create your grocery list ahead of time and make sure that it only consists of ingredients that you'll be using to prepare your meals. This will prevent you from buying on impulse or getting confused while shopping. Ideally, you want to stick to organic and whole foods with enough variety to meet your body's nutrient needs. Good carbs found in vegetables and fruit, lean protein and low GI grains are definitely the way to go to maintain a healthy and balanced diet.

Be Generous With Your Portions: Try and cook big portions, especially when it comes to dinner meals, as the leftovers will take care of lunch the following day. Just be sure to store the leftovers in the fridge overnight and warm them up before you leave so that they're nice and fresh for lunch time. Also, preparing large portions will leave you feeling satisfied after each meal and prevent overindulging at your next meal, or running to the snack bar. And it'll prevent from running out of meals before the week is done.

Have a Designated Meal Prep Day to Keep You Organised: Schedule your meal prepping time so that it falls on a particular day of the week, or you can even do it twice a week if your timetable allows. Just be sure to allocate yourself enough time to chop, cook, assemble, label and store all your meals so that it's easier to find what you're looking for during the week. Preferably 3 or more hours are enough to prepare meals for an entire week. If need be, you can also split your meal prepping to two days a week, so that you can slash your meal prepping time by half.

Use the Right Containers: The effect of good quality storage containers on your food preparing endeavours cannot be underestimated. Having the right single-serving size containers, for example, will help you stick to the right portions and prevent binge eating or feeling unsatisfied. On the other hand, BPA free, airtight and fridge friendly containers will keep your food fresh to maintain nutrients for longer. Some good quality suggestions include Tupperware, glass and stainless steel containers. Not only do they meet all the stated requirements, but they also won't melt while you're warming your food in the oven.

Another good tip is to purchase small sized containers to keep snacks, as this will prevent overindulgence during snack time, and small containers are mobile enough to take with you in a handbag when you're on the go. Lastly, glass bottles and jars are ideal for storing and travelling with your healthy smoothies and juices, and you can also use them to store things like oats, muesli and salads.

Make Meal Prep Work for You: There's a wide variety of healthy food options to choose from, so you should never feel forced to include certain health foods in your diet even if you don't like them. Rather opt for healthy versions of the foods you like, such as spiralized zucchini noodles instead of pasta, or avocado fat instead of butter. Through healthier ingredients, you can enjoy the health benefits of genuine food without compromising on taste and flavour.

Organise Your Fridge Right: When storing food in your fridge make sure to organise it in a way that will not only keep your food fresh but is also advantageous to your weight loss goals. For instance, keep the healthy selections at the front of the fridge so that it's the first thing you grab when feeling peckish, and keep unhealthy options in the back to avoid consuming them at all.

The best place for cooked foods is on the top shelves, while the fridge door is better suited for keeping foods with a long shelf life as it's the warmest place in the fridge. Also keep ethylene-producing plants such as bananas, avocados and tomatoes away from veggies with a short lifespan such as potatoes, cauliflower and spinach. On the other hand, the lower shelves provide ideal storage for foods that still need to be cooked, like chopped veggies and fruits.

3.2 Delicious and Nutritious Recipes

These easy and healthy weight loss recipes taste amazing! The collection includes tasty and simple breakfast, lunch and dinner ideas that will help you lose weight, without feeling like you need to restrict. So, if you're looking for some easy meals that will help you lose weight sustainably, while also enjoying them – this is the list for you! No need to eat bland boring food or no food at all, because you're striving to lose 10 pounds this month!

Let's start with breakfast! These are a few go-to favorite recipes for weight loss to start your day right.

Easy Overnight Oats: I guess oatmeal and overnight oats aren't a surprise to anyone who's on a weight loss journey. They're super easy to make, filling, versatile and highly nutritious.

Avocado Egg Sandwich: Craving something savory in the morning? This tasty avocado egg sandwich with spinach and other vegetables will not disappoint!

Healthy Breakfast Apple Crumble: You can make this crumble whenever you want especially when apples are in season. It's just so good! You can enjoy it for breakfast with some homemade cashew milk, but can also make a batch and have it for dessert with some ice cream.

Mediterranean Breakfast Egg Scramble: If you love Mediterranean food and are aiming to lose weight, then try scrambled eggs! They're easy to make, low in carbs and so tasty!

Let's have a look at the lunch and dinner ideas.
Mediterranean Chickpea Tuna Salad: This meal is lovely, quick and refreshing. If you've got some canned food and fresh produce you can make it in like 10 minutes.

Spicy Shrimp and Quinoa: You'll need cooked quinoa, frozen shrimp, vegetables and garlic to make this quick tasty dinner!

Ground Beef and Vegetable Skillet: One pan, vegetables, ground meat, herbs and spices are the things you need to make this amazing dinner skillet! It's low carb and you can serve it with some avocado or other fresh vegetables of choice.

Anti-Inflammatory Salmon Salad: Chronic inflammation is running high these days and weight gain is linked to it, so make this tasty super healthy salmon salad in order to reduce it.

15-Minute Spicy Shrimp Vegetable Stir-Fry: Some frozen shrimp, frozen green beans, extra vegetables, a large pan, 15 minutes and you've got yourself a nutritious flavorful dinner!

20-Minute Ground Beef and Cabbage Recipe: You'll love this ground beef and cabbage skillet!

It's few ingredients, really easy to make and you only need one pan. Plus it's so good!

Salmon Lettuce Wraps: Flavorful amazing salmon wraps with vegetables and an easy herby garlic sauce!

Ground Turkey Mushroom Soup: This ground turkey recipe is super healthy, light, satisfying and ready in about 20-30 minutes.

Healthy Chicken Recipes
These weight loss recipes with chicken are packed with protein, flavor and antioxidants to help you nourish your body.

Leftover Chicken Gyros Bowls: You have to make this gyros bowl! Even if you don't have leftover chicken, try it with whatever type of chicken or meat you enjoy – it's just so good and it's low-carb.

Creamy Chicken and Vegetables: Yes, it's another chicken recipe that can help you lose weight and it's made in one pan with lots of vegetables. It's creamy and so good!

Healthy Egg Roll In A Bowl With Chicken: If you haven't had the famous dish called "egg roll in a bowl", you just have to! Even if you're not attempting to lose weight! You'll actually start craving cabbage once you give it a go!

Easy Avocado Chicken Salad: Super filling, super flavorful avocado chicken salad with eggs, cucumbers, spinach and tomatoes. High in protein, antioxidant-rich and low in carbs – the perfect weight loss recipe!

Mediterranean Chicken Lettuce Wraps: These chicken lettuce wraps are light, yet satiating and great for meal prep too!

Mashed Avocado Chicken Salad: If you've got some shredded chicken or leftover rotisserie chicken you can make this tasty salad in like 5 minutes! Wrap it in lettuce or serve on toast for lunch or even breakfast!

Spicy Roasted Vegetable Chicken Bowls: Chicken and lots of vegetables in different shapes and colors: fresh cabbage, lettuce, dill, garlic, spicy roasted cauliflower, bell peppers and cauliflower, all come together with a tasty yogurt garlic sauce.

Chapter 4: Smart Exercise Integration

4.1 Maximizing Workouts for Weight Loss

Many types of physical activity can support weight loss by increasing the calories you burn. The amount of weight you can expect to lose may vary depending on your age, diet, and starting weight. Estimates state that around half of all American adults attempt to lose weight yearly. Exercising is one of the most common strategies employed by those trying to shed a few pounds. It burns calories, and this plays a key role in weight loss.

In addition to helping you lose weight, exercise has many other benefits, including improved mood, stronger bones and a reduced risk of many chronic diseases.

Here are the best exercises for weight loss.
Walking: Walking can be a convenient way for many beginners to exercise without feeling overwhelmed or needing to purchase equipment. It's also a lower-impact exercise, meaning it's less likely to stress your joints. According to the American Council on Exercise, a 140-pound (65-kilogram) person burns about 7.6 calories per minute walking. A 180-pound (81-kg) person burns about 9.7 calories per minute walking. A study of 20 women with obesity found that walking for 50–70 minutes 3 times per week reduced body fat and waist circumference by an average of 1.5% and 1.1 inches (2.8 cm), respectively. To get started, aim to walk for 30 minutes 3–4 times a week. You

can gradually increase the duration or frequency of your walks as you become more fit.

Jogging or Running: Although they seem similar, the key difference is that a jogging pace is generally between 4–6 mph (6.4–9.7 km/h), while a running pace is faster than 6 mph (9.7 km/h). The American Council on Exercise estimates that a 140-pound (65-kg) person burns about 10.8 calories per minute jogging and 13.2 calories per minute when running.

A 180-pound (81-kg) person burns about 13.9 calories per minute jogging and 17 calories per minute when running. Jogging and running can help burn visceral fat, commonly known as belly fat. This type of fat wraps around your internal organs and has links to various chronic diseases like heart disease and diabetes.

To get started, aim to jog for 20–30 minutes 3–4 times per week. If you find jogging or running outdoors hard on your joints, try running on softer surfaces like grass. Many treadmills have built-in cushioning, which may be easier on your joints.

Cycling: Cycling is a non-weight-bearing and low impact exercise, so it won't place much stress on your joints. The American Council on Exercise estimates that a 140-pound (65-kg) person burns about 6.4 calories per minute cycling at a speed of 10 miles per hour (MPH). A 180-pound (81-kg) person burns about 8.2 calories per minute cycling at 10 MPH. Studies have also found that people who cycle regularly have better overall fitness, increased insulin sensitivity, and a lower risk of heart disease, cancer, and death than those who don't cycle regularly. Although cycling is traditionally an outdoor activity, many gyms and fitness centers have stationary bikes that allow you to cycle while staying indoors.

Weight Training: Weight training can help build strength and promote muscle growth, raising your resting metabolic rate (RMR), or how many calories your body burns at rest. The American Council on Exercise estimates that a 140-pound (65-kg) person burns about 7.6 calories per minute of weight training. A 180-pound person burns about 9.8 calories per minute of weight training. One six month study showed that doing 11 minutes of strength-based exercises three times per week resulted in an average 7.4% increase in metabolic rate. In this study, that increase was equivalent to burning an additional 125 calories per day. Another study found that

24 weeks of weight training led to a 9% increase in men's metabolic rate, equating to burning approximately 140 more calories per day. Among women, the increase in metabolic rate was nearly 4% or 50 more calories per day.

In addition, studies have shown that your body continues to burn calories many hours after a weight-training workout, compared with aerobic exercise.

Interval Training: Interval training, more commonly known as high intensity interval training (HIIT), is a broad term for short bursts of intense exercise that alternate with recovery periods. Typically, a HIIT workout lasts 10–30 minutes and can burn many calories. One study of 9 active men found that HIIT burned 25–30% more calories per minute than other types of exercises, including weight training, cycling, and running on a treadmill. That means HIIT can help you burn more calories while exercising less. Numerous studies have shown that HIIT is especially effective at burning belly fat, which has links to many chronic diseases. To get started, choose a type of exercise, such as running, jumping, or biking, and your exercise and rest times. For example, pedal as hard as you can on a bike for 30 seconds, then pedal slowly for 1–2 minutes. Repeat this pattern for 10–30 minutes.

Swimming: The American Council on Exercise estimates that a 140-pound (65-kg) person burns about 9 calories per minute swimming at a crawl or moderate pace. A 180-pound (81-kg) person burns about 11.6 calories per minute swimming at a crawl or moderate pace. How you swim appears to affect how many calories you burn. One study on competitive swimmers found that the most calories were burned during the breaststroke, followed by the butterfly, backstroke, and freestyle.

Swimming for 60 minutes 3 times per week can significantly reduced body fat, improved flexibility, and reduced several heart disease risk factors, including high total cholesterol and blood triglycerides. Swimming is its low impact nature, meaning it's easier on your joints. This makes it a great option for people with injuries or joint pain.

Yoga: While it's not commonly considered a weight loss exercise, yoga burns a fair amount of calories and offers many additional health benefits that can promote weight loss. Women with obesity who may participate in a 90 minutes yoga sessions per week would experience greater reductions in waist circumference than those in the control group—by 1.5 inches (3.8 cm), on average. The yoga group also experienced improvements in mental and physical well-being. In fact, studies have shown that yoga can teach mindfulness and reduce stress levels. Most gyms offer yoga classes, but you can practice yoga anywhere. This includes from the comfort of your own home, as there are plenty of guided tutorials online.

Pilates: A person weighing around 140 pounds (64 kg) would burn 108 calories at a 30-minute beginner's Pilates class or 168 calories at an advanced class of the same duration.

Although Pilates may not burn as many calories as aerobic exercises like running, many people find it enjoyable, which makes it easier to stick to over time. Performing Pilates exercises for 90 minutes 3 times per week significantly reduced waist, stomach, and hip circumference, compared with a control group that did no exercise over the same period. Pilates may also reduce lower back pain and improve strength, balance, flexibility, endurance, and overall fitness. You can do Pilates at home or at one of the many gyms that offer Pilates classes.

To further boost weight loss with Pilates, combine it with a balanced diet and other forms of exercise, such as weight training or cardio.

4.2 Customizing Your Fitness Routine

Before customizing your fitness routines, there are so many things to be considered as an individual such as assessing your abilities, defining your goals, creating a customized workout plan, cardio plan and sample workout programs.

Step 1: Assessing Your Abilities

First, you need to assess your abilities. Taking your current abilities into account is the starting point of every personalized exercise plan. Here are the three questions you need to ask yourself to assess your abilities.

- What is your body composition?
- What are your movement abilities?
- What is your current level of fitness?

Now, let's break them down individually and look at how they will affect your workout plan.

What is Your Body Composition?

In this context, body composition refers to your ratio of lean muscle to body fat. We recommend that you check in on your current body composition before you start your workout plan. Taking into account your current composition can help you establish your goals and give you a way to track progress. If your fitness goals are rooted in body composition, take a photo of yourself or get an Inbody analysis that you can refer back to.

What are Your Movement Abilities?
Think back to the last time you worked out. What movements could you easily do and what movements were difficult or even painful? Write your answers down, as this information will come in handy when you pick exact exercises later on. For the best results, have a professional fitness coach assess your movement.

What is Your Current Level of Fitness?

The key to getting results from your workout plan is finding the sweet spot of difficulty. You don't want something too easy or too tough. The perfect amount of exercise will challenge you but just enough to where you can remain consistent. So think back to different workouts you've done. What has been too easy and what was too tough? Write this down because your answer will dictate how long your weight training and cardio workouts will be and what they will consist of.

Assess Your Resources

For the last part of your assessment, take stock of your resources.

- How many days a week can you work out?
- How much time can you work out a day?

- What fitness equipment do you have access to?
- How much can you spend on food?

You need to understand your resources. They will have a direct impact on your personalized workout plan.

Step 2: Defining Your Goals

Now you know your starting point, it's time to define your goals. First, start by asking yourself why you want to work out? Then, don't settle for the surface answer. Dig deeper into your truer motivations. For example, if your goal is to lose weight, then why is this important to you? Is it to be an example for your family? Or is it to reach your full potential as a human? Whatever it is, understanding your true motivation will make it easier to stick to your personalized workout plan.

Next, create a SMART goal.

Step 3: Creating a Customized Workout Plan

With the information from the assessment and your goals in hand, it is time to create your personalized workout plan. A balanced workout plan for general health should include a combination of weight training (resistance training) and cardio (aerobic training). We like to combine these two types of exercise because resistance training creates a great metabolic advantage, while a strong aerobic system will help you recover faster and boost your immune system.

Two Types of Workout Plans

We will cover how to create two personalized workout plans: one for beginners and one for more advanced individuals. If you don't know where you fall, then start with the beginner program. Even advanced individuals will see results.

The Beginner Weekly Training Split

If you are a beginner, exercise between 4 and 5 times a week. On 2 to 3 of those days, do full-body weight training workouts. On the other days, do sustainable cardio workouts. These days may be in the gym, but can also be activities outside the gym, such as walks, hikes, bike rides, and playing outdoor sports. Alternate between resistance and aerobic training throughout the week.

Here's a sample for the beginner weekly split:

- Monday: Weight Training (Full body)
- Tuesday: Walk, Hike, or Bike
- Wednesday: Weight Training (Full body)
- Thursday: Walk, Hike, or Bike
- Friday: Weight Training (Full body)
- Saturday: Active rest day
- Sunday: Active rest day

The Advanced Training Split

If you are advanced, then you'll likely exercise between 4 and 6 days a week. On 2-4 of those days, you can lift weights. Split those training days up between upper and lower body days. On the other days, do sustainable cardio workouts and stay active by walking on your non-training days.

Here's a same for the advanced weekly split:

- Monday: Weight Training (Upper body)
- Tuesday: Cardio (Rowing, Biking, or Walking)
- Wednesday: Weight Training (Lower body)
- Thursday: Weight Training (Upper body)
- Friday: Cardio (Rowing, Biking, or Walking)
- Saturday: Weight Training (Lower body)
- Sunday: Active rest day

Now that you have the weekly split, let's lay in the exercises for each day. For weight training, six movement patterns make up all of the exercises you find in the gym; squat, bend, lunge, push, pull, and core. If you are a beginner, train 5-6 of these patterns every time you workout.

If you are more advanced, divide these movement patterns up into upper (push, pull, and core) and lower (squat, bend, lunge, and core) body exercises. Then choose one exercise from each pattern.

When writing exercises for a training day, order them from the most complex to least complex. Multi-joint compound movements come first in the training day. Examples include the squat, bench press, and the deadlift. Simple-single joint movements come next. Examples include shoulder lateral raises, bicep curls, and leg extensions.

For example:

A) Bench Press, @3010, 8-10 reps x 3 sets; rest 60 seconds

B1) Bent Over Barbell Row, @2021, 8-10 reps x 3 sets; rest 60 seconds

B2) Landmine Press, @2021 8-10 reps x 3 sets; rest 60 seconds

C1) Seated Single Arm Bicep Curl, @2021 8-10 reps x 3 sets; rest 60 seconds

C2) Chest Supported Cable Tricep Pushdown, @2021 10-12 reps x 3 sets; rest 60 seconds

Choose Rep Ranges, Sets, and Rest Time

When choosing rep ranges for beginners, we prefer anywhere between 8-15 reps. This rep range is the best for developing your motor control and muscle endurance. A common number of sets for beginners is 2-4. As you become more advanced, you can perform lower repetitions at higher loads to develop strength endurance and eventually, maximal contractions. Lastly, don't forget your rest time. While it's popular to hit exercises back to back for maximum intensity, taking breaks between exercises is important. Rest allows you to recover and then perform the same exercise at a similar intensity.

Quality over Quantity

When you're weight training, the goal is to learn the movement patterns and create tension in the muscle. To see the best results, you need to keep this in mind and focus on the quality of movement over quantity. Reps with poor quality and tension will reinforce bad patterns and be ineffective. 20 really good reps are better than 100 really bad ones.

Step 4: Creating a Cardio Workout Plan
Cardio workouts are sustainable aerobic exercise performed for an extended period of time. Cardio has a host of health benefits including improved immune function, cognitive function, and quicker recovery. To create a cardio workout choose a form of exercise. We like walking, biking, rowing, hiking, and running. Next, pick a duration or distance and go at a pace that you can easily complete. Start by completing the exercise for the determined duration or distance. Then over time start increasing the duration or distance. Slowly increasing the workout over time will ensure that your cardio progression

stays sustainable, which is the key to building your aerobic system.

Sample Cardio Workout Progression:

- Week 1: Walk for 20 Minutes or bike 4 miles
- Week 2: Walk for 30 Minutes or bike 5 miles
- Week 3: Walk for 40 Minutes or bike 6 miles
- Week 4: Walk for 50 Minutes or bike 7 miles

This may seem simple, but it is highly effective. To build your cardiovascular fitness, you need to do slow and easy movement that is easily repeatable. Give it a try and you will be surprised by the base you can build.

Step 5: Sample Workouts Programs

Sample Beginner Full Body Workout Plan:

A1) Kettlebell Romanian Deadlift @3030, 8-10 reps x 3 sets; rest 60 seconds

A2) Dumbbell Bench Press @2111, 8-10 reps x 3 sets ; rest 60 seconds

B1) Goblet Squat @3311, 8-10 reps x 3 sets; rest 60 seconds

B2) Seated Lat Pull Down @3012, 8-10 reps x 3 sets; rest 60 seconds

C) Banded Dead Bug @3030, 10-12 reps x 3 sets; rest 60 seconds

Sample Advanced Upper Body Workout Program

A) Weighted Pull Up @1221, 3-4 reps x 4 sets x 3 sets; rest 2-3 minutes

B1) Seated Dumbbell Press @2121, 5-6 reps x 3 sets; rest 90 seconds

B2) Single Arm Landmine Row @2121, 5-6 reps x 3 sets; rest 2 minutes

C1) Dumbbell Fly @2121, 8-10 x 3 sets; rest 90 seconds

C2) Plate Loaded Deadbug 10 per leg x 3 sets; rest 90 seconds

Lower Body Training Day:

A) Romanian Deadlift @1120, 3-4 reps x 4 sets; rest 2-3 minutes

B) Front Rack Split Squat @2121, 5-6 reps x 3 sets; rest 2 minutes

C1) Kettlebell Front Rack Wall Sit, 30-45 seconds x 3 sets, rest 90 seconds
C2) Weighted Front Plank, 60 seconds x 3 sets, rest 90 seconds

Chapter 5: Mindful Eating and Emotional Balance

5.1 Mindful Eating Practices

The world is filled with fast-paced meals and distractions, eating mindfully can enhance your weight loss journey. It's not just about what you eat but how you eat. Let's look at the mindful eating practices to loose weight.

Presence at the Plate: Begin by bringing your full attention to the dining table. Avoid distractions like screens or multitasking. Engage your senses—observe the colors, textures, and aromas of your food.

Eating with Intention: Set an intention for your meal. Whether it's nourishing your body with energy for the day or savoring the flavors of each bite, having a purpose brings mindfulness to your eating experience.

Slow and Savored Bites: Chew your food slowly, savoring each bite. Not only does this enhance the enjoyment of your meal, but it also allows your body to recognize signals of fullness, preventing overeating.

Recognizing Hunger and Fullness: Learn to listen to your body's signals. Distinguish between physical hunger and emotional cravings. Mindful eating encourages you to eat when you're hungry and stop when you're satisfied.

Cultivating Gratitude: Take a moment to express gratitude for your meal. Acknowledge the effort that went into preparing the food and the nourishment it provides. This simple practice can shift your perspective on eating.

Identifying Emotional Triggers: Mindful eating involves recognizing emotional triggers for eating. Whether it's stress, boredom, or celebration, understanding your emotional relationship with food is a key step toward mindful practices.

Portion Awareness: Be conscious of portion sizes. Mindful eating isn't about deprivation but about understanding what your body needs. Recognize when you've had enough and honor your body's signals.

Logging Your Experience: Consider keeping a food journal. Record not just what you eat but also your emotions and physical sensations. This reflection can provide valuable insights into your eating patterns.

Mindful Grocery Shopping: Extend mindfulness to your grocery shopping. Make intentional choices, opt for whole foods, and savor the process of selecting items that contribute to your well-being.

Creating Rituals: Establish mealtime rituals that bring joy and mindfulness. Whether it's lighting a candle, playing soft music, or setting a beautiful table, these rituals enhance your eating experience.

5.2 Managing Stress and Emotional Eating

Stress and weight loss have a complicated relationship. At times, high stress can lead to unhealthy and often-temporary weight loss caused by skipping meals or being overly active. Frequently, weight lost in this fashion usually returns. Chronic and uncontrollable stress can undermine your efforts to eat healthy, exercise, sleep, and develop healthy habits. And, unhealthy weight-loss patterns usually intensifies the stress.

In fact, stress can create many physical challenges and changes in your body if not managed properly. For example, when you're stressed you might find yourself eating more junk food, or "stress eating," even when you're not hungry. Stress can also slow your metabolism and make it harder to burn fat, particularly belly fat. Unhealthy stress can also lower your self-regulation, making it harder to exercise and maintain healthy habits. Sleep and stress are often connected in a vicious cycle: stress causes sleep loss, making you feel more vulnerable to it, which intensifies your sleeplessness. Luckily, you can develop the skills to help lower stress when it's unnecessary.

Make Stress an Ally

While most people believe that stress is seriously harmful to their health, it turns out that your "stress mindset," or how you think about stress, influences whether your reaction to it will impact you positively or negatively. When you think about stress as your ally, rather than your enemy, you can train yourself to experience more of the positive effects of the stress response. For example, healthy stress causes you to stick to your exercise routine, your meal plan, and it is what triggers you to even bother getting out of bed in the morning. Your heart rate naturally accelerates from stressors—this means that your blood vessels relax, inflammation decreases, and the pumping mimics exercise, which helps to boost your cardiovascular health.

Although stress can be good, it's also important that you know how to recognize when your stress levels are unhealthy. By developing the skills to activate your relaxation response, you can lower your stress levels and stay in control. Once you learn different relaxation response skills, choose one to practice every day for at least a week. Like any skill, you will get better with practice, so it's important to practice these skills "to calm you down," even when they aren't needed. In the same way, you wouldn't want to only practice your swimming skills during a rescue.

Reframe Threats to Challenges

Next time you're in a stressful situation, you can choose how to interpret it. Is it a true threat? Is this something that will bring you down? Or you might view the threat as a challenge and think, "This is an opportunity to learn something." It's your chance to prove that you have the resources to deal effectively with this situation. Shifting the lens from threat to challenge—from adversity to opportunity—can open-up your perception.

Embrace Anxiety

Nervousness can feel unpleasant, and the emotion and physical embodiment of anxiety often becomes a source of stress. Many have been taught to "relax away the symptoms" when they're feeling stressed. However, research shows that trying to calm down can negatively impact your performance, so reinterpret your anxiety as excitement. Tell yourself that the sensations you feel are helping your mind and body prepare, rather than they being a sign that you can't handle what's going on. The reframe will help you to boost your performance and enable you to feel more confident and composed.

Relax When Needed

Recovery is essential to help you stay robust while you cope with stress. When your stress response is chronically on overdrive, it can drain your energy and make you more susceptible to illness and injury. Use mind-body techniques such as deep breathing, imagery, and progressive muscle relaxation to activate the "rest and digest" system to balance out your fight-or-flight response. Also, prioritize sleep because it helps you feel armed and at-the-ready to manage your stress.

Connect to Bigger-Than-Self Goals

It can be a challenge to find meaning in day-to-day hassles like the ones you experience at work and home. When you're feeling burned out, turn your self-focused goals into "bigger-than-self" ones by connecting to those values and life aspirations that matter most. What's driving you? How will a healthier lifestyle contribute to the world and those around you? What kind of positive impact can you make? Is it honorably serving your nation? If you have children, is it raising them to be compassionate? Focus on something larger than yourself.

Exercise More

The energy you feel when overly stressed can be overwhelming. As you notice the effects of stress in your body, such as your heart rate increasing, you can unknowingly intensify those sensations. However, you can put that energy to use by exercising more. Exercise can help you calm your nerves, distract you from your stressful thoughts, and assist you in losing weight.

Sometimes the strongest food cravings hit when you're at your weakest point emotionally. You may turn to food for comfort — consciously or unconsciously — when facing a difficult problem, feeling stressed or even feeling bored. Emotional eating can sabotage your weight-loss efforts. It often leads to eating too much — especially too much of high-calorie, sweet and fatty foods. The good news is that if you're prone to emotional eating, you can take steps to regain control of your eating habits and get back on track with your weight-loss goals. To help stop emotional eating, try these tips:

Keep a Food Diary: Write down what you eat, how much you eat, when you eat, how you're feeling when you eat and how hungry you are. Over time, you might see patterns that reveal the connection between mood and food.

Tame Your Stress. If stress contributes to your emotional eating, try a stress management technique, such as yoga, meditation or deep breathing.

Have a Hunger Reality Check: Is your hunger physical or emotional? If you ate just a few hours ago and don't have a rumbling stomach, you're probably not hungry. Give the craving time to pass.

Get Support: You're more likely to give in to emotional eating if you lack a good support network. Lean on family and friends or consider joining a support group.

Fight Boredom: Instead of snacking when you're not hungry, distract yourself and substitute a healthier behavior. Take a walk, watch a movie, play with your cat, listen to music, read, surf the internet or call a friend.

Take Away Temptation: Don't keep hard-to-resist comfort foods in your home. And if you feel angry or blue, postpone your trip to the grocery store until you have your emotions in check.

Don't Deprive Yourself: When trying to lose weight, you might limit calories too much, eat the same foods repeatedly and banish treats. This may just serve to increase your food cravings, especially in response to emotions. Eat satisfying amounts of healthier foods, enjoy an occasional treat and get plenty of variety to help curb cravings.

Snack Healthy: If you feel the urge to eat between meals, choose a healthy snack, such as fresh fruit, vegetables with low-fat dip, nuts or unbuttered popcorn. Or try lower calorie versions of your favorite foods to see if they satisfy your craving.

Learn from Setbacks: If you have an episode of emotional eating, forgive yourself and start fresh the next day. Try to learn from the experience and make a plan for how you can prevent it in the future. Focus on the positive changes you're making in your eating habits and give yourself credit for making changes that'll lead to better health.

Chapter 6: Establishing Sustainable Habits

6.2 Forming Healthy Eating Patterns

Many people achieve short term weight loss through drastic measures such as fasting or cutting out certain foods which can lead to feelings of deprivation and discouragement. The weight may come off at first, but when old habits return, so does the weight. Here are healthy eating habits to lose weight that can help improve your nutrition without giving up your favorite foods, enhance your health, protect your mental well-being, and keep the weight off for good!

Avoid Drinking Your Calories: Popular beverages like juice, soda, alcoholic drinks, and some coffee drinks can be loaded with calories from added sugars. Chewing food takes time, but swigging back a high-calorie or alcoholic drink is easy, and before you know it, you're asking for a refill. Because of that, high-calorie beverages can hamper your weight loss progress. Ultra-processed beverages such as soda are also more likely to cause inflammation and lead to chronic disease. Swapping a soda for a diet version is a solution some use to lose weight. However, diet sodas and other zero-calorie drinks are sometimes sweetened with an artificial sweetener called sucralose. Opting for a diet beverage can be alright in moderation, but it is best to avoid drinking them frequently. A study found that regular sucralose intake led to a higher motivation to eat and more calories consumed. It's best not to rely on sucralose-sweetened drinks as a go-to weight loss solution. Instead, drink water most of the time, which will keep your body well hydrated. You can keep it interesting by adding berries or citrus slices to infuse water or herbs like mint or basil.

Pre-Load Your Meals With Salads: Eating a salad before your entree has many benefits. First, a salad is an opportunity to get some vegetable servings into your day. Vegetables are a cornerstone of a healthy diet because they're high in fiber, vitamins, minerals, and antioxidants, and low in calories, fat, and carbohydrates. Another benefit of a pre-meal salad is that fiber can help you feel full faster and could curb how much you eat when it's time for your meal. In turn, you may consume fewer calories, which over time could decrease your weight.

Practice Mindful Eating: It's not uncommon to eat while you also scroll your newsfeed or get some work done. Mindful eating helps you focus on your meal, free of distractions, so that you can focus on enjoying your meal——the taste, smell, texture, and visual appeal. That way, you're more in tune with your body while attentive to your chewing, swallowing, hunger, and fullness cues. Research shows that your environment can influence how much or how little you eat, so mindful eating lets your body take back control and allows you to be thoughtful about when you're done eating.

Avoid Eating Late: Whether it's salty chips or a bowl of ice cream, late-night snacks may interfere with your weight loss goals. The timing of your meals matters. According to research, late-night eating can disrupt sleep patterns, which may also influence appetite. Eating fiber and protein-rich meals during the day can help lessen the desire to eat late in the evenings.

Choose Whole Grains Most of the Time: Make half of your daily grain intake whole grains. Whole grain seeds or kernels have three nutritious parts – bran, germ, and endosperm. Whole grains are rich in B vitamins, protein, fiber, healthy fats, minerals, and complex carbohydrates. Pasta, white bread, and crackers are examples of refined grains. The bran and germ are lost through the processing of refined grains, making them less nutritious foods. Whole grains are a better option because they're more likely to fill you up with their fiber-rich contents, which can help with weight loss.

Keep Your Meals Balanced: Eating meals that offer balance, variety, and color can significantly impact weight loss. The key is to eat multiple food groups at once. If you've ever eaten a muffin for breakfast, you may have noticed a surge of energy followed by a crash. After an hour or less, your hunger pangs begin, and you're ready to eat again. Eating just a muffin is not offering your body enough nutrition to support sustained energy and spur weight loss. Depending on the size of the muffin, you may consider cutting it in half and adding hard boiled eggs and fresh raspberries to your breakfast. You're adding protein to create a healthy meal that will keep you full for longer, help balance your blood sugars, and promote weight loss. Adding fruit like fresh raspberries gives you fiber and loads of vitamins and minerals essential to your body. A good rule of thumb for balancing meals is to fill half your plate with non-starchy vegetables, one-quarter with fruit, and the remaining one-quarter with lean protein.

Don't Overly Restrict Yourself: Following fad diets or diet plans that are strict about your eating habits can cause out-of-control eating behaviors and affect your mental health. Restrictive eating can be dangerous and mirror eating disorders.

Mind Your Portion Sizes: Consistently eating large portions can provide more calories than you need, leading to weight gain over time. Practicing portion control is more important than ever because restaurant portions have become progressively larger. If you are tempted to finish these portions, try to listen to your body's satiety cues and ask for a to-go box to enjoy the rest of your meal for lunch or dinner the next day. To avoid eating more than you need at one time, try eating smaller portions to lose and maintain a healthy weight, paying attention to your body's hunger and fullness cues to adjust as needed.

Embrace Your Inner Chef: Restaurants and fast food joints are infamous for producing foods that offer more calories in a meal than you need in an entire day. The solution? Cooking more at home. Consider the things you like to eat out and try to whip up a healthier version at home. The best part about cooking at home is that you're in control of what you make, how you cook the food, and what ingredients you add. While it's still possible to eat out and still lose weight, cooking at home more often puts you in a better position to master your health goals.

Try Meal Prepping: Meal prep is a great way to give yourself the gift of healthy home cooked meals. When you think of meal prep, you might imagine a row of perfectly portioned meal containers ready to go in the fridge. But, there are multiple types of meal prepping, and it's best to pick one that suits your lifestyle. Some people prep meals ahead of time that they can grab and take to work, and others may meal prep by making slow cooker freezer meals. Meal prep can be as easy as prepping ingredients ahead of time, like chopping up vegetables so they're ready for a Friday night stir-fry or boiling eggs for breakfast the next morning. Whatever it may be, make meal prepping work for you to ensure that you have healthy meals to eat throughout the week. Meal prepping can also help in controlling food portion sizes, making the amount you eat at each meal more consistent.

Introduce Healthy Fats to Your Diet: Fats have gained a healthier reputation in recent years. Still, it's essential to watch your saturated fat intake for overall health and choose healthy fat sources more often. Healthy fats, or unsaturated fats, may help with weight loss by increasing satiety which suppresses your appetite. Healthy fats for weight loss include avocados, nuts, nut butter, full-fat yogurt, and salmon. You can eat mashed avocados in a dip with fresh veggies or enjoy full-fat yogurt with cinnamon and sliced bananas for dessert. It is important to note that too much fat, especially saturated fats, can hinder weight loss efforts and even lead to medical conditions such as high blood pressure or increased cholesterol levels.

Keep Healthy Food Accessible: Opening a bag of snacks takes less effort than peeling an orange. It sounds trivial, but access can make a difference in a person's food choice. Make eating nutritious foods a simple decision by pre-cutting fruit and vegetables and placing them in view. You can leave fruits like apples and bananas in a fruit bowl on the counter and put pre-cut produce in a clear container, that way, you see them each time you open your fridge. Consider keeping nuts, dried fruit, and seeds in see-through canisters so they're easily accessible for a nutrient-rich snack. By doing so you will be able to better incorporate a variety of foods and food groups into your daily diet.

Carry Healthy Snacks With You: Packing healthy snacks on the go is a way to set yourself up for weight loss success, plus it helps you avoid swinging through the drive-thru on an empty stomach. A lunch bag with an ice pack helps to keep healthy snacks like cheese sticks, yogurt, and hummus cold. Non-perishables are great to take along with you or stow away in your car. Nuts, seeds, rice cakes, bison jerky, peanut butter packs, and protein bars are some ideas.

Start Your Day With Plants: According to the Centers for Disease Control, only 9% of Americans are eating enough vegetables and 12% eat enough fruit. Research tells us that plant-based and vegetarian diets are linked with lower body weights, and these diets are plentiful in fruits, vegetables, legumes, nuts, seeds, and whole grains. Your average American breakfast contains fatty meats like sausages and bacon, calorie-laden gravies, and sugary foods like muffins, syrups, donuts, and croissants. While fruit is a standard breakfast item, other plant foods like vegetables, nuts, seeds, and beans are typically eaten later in the day. You can increase your intake of plant foods and reap their countless benefits by enjoying them at your morning meal. Consider adding leafy greens or other veggies to scrambled eggs, topping a yogurt parfait with sliced almonds or sunflower seeds, or adding a side of black beans or diced sweet potatoes to a breakfast wrap.

6.2 Daily Routines for Long-term Success

Hop on the Scale: Weighing yourself first thing in the morning after you pee is more accurate than checking later in the day. What you eat and drink later on can change the results. That visual reminder of your weight each morning can help you stick to your healthy eating plan the rest of the day or week.

Drink a Glass (or 2) of Water: One or two glasses of plain H2O before you eat breakfast may help you lose weight. Water has no calories, but it's satisfying and curbs your appetite, so you may not want to eat such a big breakfast afterward. It also stimulates your metabolismto help you burn calories.

Work Out Before Breakfast: Do some moderate exercise before you sit down to eat in the mornings. Working out on an empty stomach actually helps you get better results from exercise. Prebreakfast sweat sessions can help you burn more of your body's fat for fuel.

Eat a High-Protein Breakfast: This nutrient may help you lose weight because it makes you feel fuller longer after you eat. It's also harder for your body to store it as excess fat. Another perk of protein: Your body uses more calories to break it down than it uses for carbs or fat. Go for protein-rich breakfasts, such as an egg and turkey sausage on whole wheat toast or a Greek yogurt smoothie with peanut butter and berries.

Make a Meal Plan for the Day: Every morning, write up a quick list of what you'll eat that day. Planning meals ahead of time can help you choose lower-calorie foods. If you've already decided what to eat for your day's snacks and meals, you may be less likely to reach for high-calorie convenience foods like fast-food burgers or fries.

Get Some Sun: Some sunlight on your skin can actually help you burn a little bit more body fat. Research shows that people who soak up a few rays in the morning tend to have a lower body-mass index (BMI), or a leaner, slimmer physique, than people who step out in the sun later in the day.

Use Measuring Cups and Spoons: It's easy to supersize portions that pack more calories than you need without even knowing it. Keep measuring cups and spoons where you typically dish out breakfast. Measure foods like cereal or milk before you place them in the bowl so you serve yourself the right amount.

Practice Mindfulness: Slow down and think about what you're eating. Appreciate the smell, look, and taste of even a simple breakfast. Don't watch TV or scroll through social media when you eat in the morning: just breathe, relax, and enjoy a peaceful meal. This practice could help you eat less and lose weight.

Use a Juice Glass: Most standard drinking glasses are far larger than a serving of juice. That makes it easy to consume more than you should. And many fruit juices have as much sugar in them as a can of soda. But they also have lots of vitamins and minerals that are great for you as you start your day. To pour a more sensible portion, use a small juice glass.

Don't Dress Up Your Coffee: Do you have your dessert in your coffee cup each morning? Specialty coffees with lots of added sugar, cream, or flavored syrups can add up to more than 500 calories each. Use skim milk or sugar-free flavors instead. Or try green tea for a morning jolt. It has catechins, nutrients that may promote weight loss.

Chapter 7: Overcoming Challenges and Plateaus

7.1 Conquering Weight Loss Plateaus

You've been working hard to follow a healthy, low-calorie diet and improve your exercise habits. And your rewards have been watching your weight go down and feeling better. Now, however, for no reason you can identify, the scale has stopped budging. You've hit a weight-loss plateau. Don't get discouraged. It's typical for weight loss to slow and even stall. By understanding what causes a weight-loss plateau, you can decide how to respond and avoid backsliding on your new healthy habits.

What is a Weight-Loss Plateau?

A weight-loss plateau is when your weight stops changing. Being stuck at a weight-loss plateau eventually happens to everyone who tries to lose weight. Even so, most people are surprised when it happens to them because they're still eating carefully and exercising regularly. The frustrating reality is that even well-planned weight-loss efforts can stall.

What Causes a Weight-Loss Plateau?

During the first few weeks of losing weight, a rapid drop is typical. In part, this is because when you initially cut calories, the body gets needed energy by releasing its stores of glycogen. Glycogen is a type of carbohydrate found in the muscles and the liver. Glycogen is partly made of water. So when glycogen is burned for energy, it releases water, resulting in weight loss that's mostly water. But this effect is temporary. As you lose weight, you lose some muscle along with fat. Muscle helps keep up the rate at which you burn calories (metabolism). So as you lose weight, your metabolism declines, causing you to burn fewer calories than you did at your heavier weight. Your slower metabolism will slow your weight loss, even if you eat the same number of calories that helped you lose weight. When the calories you burn equal the calories you eat, you reach a plateau. To lose more weight, you need to either increase your physical activity or decrease the calories you eat. Using the same approach that worked at first may maintain your weight loss, but it won't lead to more weight loss.

How Can You Conquer a Weight-Loss Plateau?

When you reach a plateau, you may have lost all of the weight you will lose on your current diet and exercise plan. Ask yourself if you're satisfied with your current weight or if you want to lose more. If you want to lose more weight, you'll need to adjust your weight-loss program.

If you're committed to losing more weight, try these tips for getting past the plateau:

Reassess Your Habits: Look back at your food and activity records. Make sure you haven't loosened the rules. For example, look at whether you've been having larger portions, eating more processed foods or getting less exercise. Research suggests that off-and-on loosening of rules contributes to plateaus.

Cut More Calories: Further cut your daily calories, provided this doesn't put you below 1,200 calories. Fewer than 1,200 calories a day may not be enough to keep you from constant hunger, which increases your risk of overeating.

Rev Up Your Workout: Get at least 150 minutes of moderate aerobic activity or 75 minutes of vigorous aerobic activity a week, or a combination of moderate and vigorous activity. Guidelines suggest that you spread out this exercise during the course of a week. For even greater health benefit and to assist with weight loss or maintaining weight loss, at least 300 minutes a week is recommended. Adding exercises such as weightlifting to increase your muscle mass will help you burn more calories.

Pack More Activity into Your Day: Think outside the gym. Increase your general physical activity throughout the day. For example, walk more and use your car less, do more yardwork, or do vigorous spring cleaning. Any physical activity will help you burn more calories.

7.2 Strategies for Consistent Progress

It's important to continue making progress after you've overcome a weight-loss plateau. Here are some strategies that can help you do that:

Continue Tracking Your Progress: This can help you see how far you've come and how much further you have to go.

Celebrate Your Successes: Every little bit of progress counts, so don't forget to celebrate your victories.

Don't Get Complacent: Just because you've overcome a plateau doesn't mean you can slack off. Keep up the good work!

Challenge Yourself: If you feel like you've hit a plateau again, it's important to analyze what might be causing it. It could be a number of things, like not enough variety in your workouts, not enough rest and recovery, or not challenging yourself enough.

Once you've identified the cause of the plateau, you can work on addressing it. For example, if you're not getting enough variety in your workouts, try mixing things up by adding new exercises or new equipment. If you're not resting enough, make sure to schedule in some rest days and focus on recovery. And if you're not challenging yourself enough, try adding some intensity

Join a Community: This can be online or in person. Having a community of like-minded people can be a great source of support and motivation.

If you're reading this book, Trim and Thrive, you may also be interested in my book on Alzheimer's disease and prenatal fitness. Tap the links above to read them.

Thank you for purchasing my book. I'd really appreciate it if you could take a moment to leave a review. Your feedback will help me improve and make my next book even better. I'm always looking forward to improving, so please do not hold back! Thank you for your time and support.